HIIT

Beginner's Guide to Hiit & Rapid Weight Loss

(How to Achieve the Body of Your Dreams With High Intensity)

Charles Harris

Published by John Kembrey

Charles Harris

All Rights Reserved

HIIT: Beginner's Guide to Hiit & Rapid Weight Loss (How to Achieve the Body of Your Dreams With High Intensity)

ISBN 978-1-77485-124-1

All rights reserved. No part of this guide may be reproduced in any form without permission in writing from the publisher except in the case of brief quotations embodied in critical articles or reviews.

Legal & Disclaimer

The information contained in this book is not designed to replace or take the place of any form of medicine or professional medical advice. The information in this book has been provided for educational and entertainment purposes only.

The information contained in this book has been compiled from sources deemed reliable, and it is accurate to the best of the Author's knowledge; however, the Author cannot guarantee its accuracy and validity and cannot be held liable for any errors or omissions. Changes are periodically made to this book. You must consult your doctor or get professional medical advice before using any of the suggested remedies, techniques, or information in this book.

Upon using the information contained in this book, you agree to hold harmless the Author from and against any damages, costs, and expenses, including any legal fees potentially resulting from the application of any of the information provided by this guide. This disclaimer applies to any damages or injury caused by the use and application, whether directly or indirectly, of any advice or information presented, whether for breach of contract, tort, negligence, personal injury, criminal intent, or under any other cause of action.

You agree to accept all risks of using the information presented inside this book. You need to consult a professional medical practitioner in order to ensure you are both able and healthy enough to participate in this program.

Table of Contents

CHAPTER 1: PREPARING FOR HIIT 1

CHAPTER 2: WHAT IS HIIT? 16

CHAPTER 3: WHAT IS HIGH-INTENSITY INTERVAL TRAINING? 32

CHAPTER 4: TYPES OF HIIT 52

CHAPTER 5: WEEKLY TRAININGS TO GET STRONGER, FASTER, LIGHTER 58

CHAPTER 6: HIIT WORKOUTS FOR THE HOME 85

CHAPTER 7: HIIT MYTHS 100

CHAPTER 8: MIX HIIT WORKOUTS 103

CHAPTER 9: GETTING STARTED 111

CHAPTER 10: PLANNING THE TIMING OF YOUR HIGH-INTENSITY INTERVAL WORKOUT 119

CHAPTER 11: SAMPLE WORKOUT 126

CHAPTER 12: WAYS TO IMPLEMENT THE LAW OF ATTRACTION 132

CHAPTER 13: NUTRITION WITH HIIT 143

CHAPTER 14: RECOVERING FROM HIIT 147

CHAPTER 15: ENZYME ADAPTATION 153

CHAPTER 16: HOME HIIT EXERCISES 157

CHAPTER 17: MORE ON HIIT NUTRITION 166

CHAPTER 18: CATECHOLAMINES RESPONSE TO SPRINT INTERVAL TRAINING.. 170

CHAPTER 19: HIIT FOR FAT LOSS AND MUSCLE GAIN..... 181

CONCLUSION.. 190

Chapter 1: Preparing For Hiit

In the previous chapter, we learned that HIIT requires you to do high-intensity workouts. Most people new to this system however, are not aware of what high-intensity means or how workout intensity can be measured.

How do you measure workout intensity?

Workout intensity can be measured in many ways. In this book however, we will only focus on two methods.

Using a heart rate monitor

The first method can be used when measuring the intensity of cardio workouts. In this method, you use a heart rate monitor while you do your workout. You will reach the highest intensity level of activity if your heart reaches 90 beats per minute. You should slow down your workout when you reach this point.

If you have a heart monitor, you may also use it in measuring the intensity of your other workouts. If lifting weights makes your heart pound, you may also use the device to measure the intensity of this type of workout.

Using a personalized scale

If you do not have a heart rate monitor, you need to create your own scale of measuring physical exhaustion. You will use this scale to assess the intensity or level of difficulty of a workout move. Your intensity scale has a lowest level of one and a highest of five.

Level 1 intensity activity is similar to sitting on a chair. In this level, you are not exerting any effort at all. Activities of level 5 intensity are the highest level of

exhaustion possible. After doing these types of activities, you can no longer continue to work out and your muscles are too sore to be useful. When you do these types of activities, you have no choice but to rest.
As you become more fit, your limit also becomes higher. A person who has never lifted weights in his life will find 5 lbs. dumbbells challenging. However, as he trains using these dumbbells and improves his stamina and strength, his maximum weight limit also increases. He may move on from using 5 lbs. dumbbells to 15 lbs. in one or two months.

The same goes with every other exercise. As you do more of certain workout moves, it becomes easier for you to do them. Your body becomes more efficient in spending energy as you do them. You will no longer be easily exhausted after doing them.

Because of this, the intensity of a workout move varies per person. A runner may assess sprints as level 3 in the intensity scale while a strongman may assess it at 5 because he is not used to doing it. On the other hand, the strongman may grade fast-paced squats as a 2 while the same runner may grade it as a 5.

Learning the levels

Here are the levels of exhaustion that you may get from working out:

1 – Not exerting any effort / resting state

2 – Light workout / a short, slow-paced jog

3 – Moderate workout / Jogging for 30 minutes

4 – Heavy workout / Doing 10 reps bench press of your maximum weight limit

5 – Point of maximum exhaustion

Doing the running test

You can test your stamina in all the workout moves that you want to do. You can start by checking how fast you become exhausted when running. You can check your running performance by running a mile in the fastest time. Professional athletes regularly run 5-minute miles. Some can even break the 4-minute mile regularly in competitions.

Beginners in running however, take around 10-15 minutes to finish a mile. You should run a mile as fast as you can and check your time. Let's say you finish in 10 minute and you are extremely exhausted after your run. You are so exhausted that you need to sit down to catch your breath. This may mean that a 10-minute per mile pace is your level 4. This can be converted to roughly 6 miles per hour. You can go faster if you just sprint for shorter distances. Your sprint will be your level 5.

When using running in an HIIT circuit, you may warm up with a level 2 pace, equivalent to a slow jog. You can then do a sprint for 100 meters in a track. After that, you can then go to your comfortable jogging pace, which is your level 3. After half a minute in this pace, you can then go back to a sprint. You can do this for 15 minutes.

Though this may sound easy, this routine can be exhausting for a beginner. You should adjust your HIIT routine according to the types of workouts that you are doing.

Choosing a workout type

Now that you know how to measure the intensity of workouts, the next step is to choose the right types of workouts to include in your routine.

If you go to online forums that discuss HIIT, you will notice that people have integrated almost all forms of workouts to HIIT. It started out as a modified cardio workout routine. Now, people are using HIIT principles with weights, calisthenics and even sports routines. HIIT is a flexible system, which can be applied to any group of workout moves.

When doing HIIT, you are in control of what to include in your workouts. You may also copy the workout routines of people who post their HIIT routine online. You should make sure however, that you are copying from people with roughly the same fitness level as you. When selecting the types of workouts that you should include in your routine, you should consider your workout goals.

If you want to lose weight, you should use HIIT principles with a combination of cardio workouts and calisthenics. If you want to gain muscle while you are losing weight, you should probably add some free-weight or resistance band training to the mix. You are in complete control with what you want to add to your routine.

HIIT Workout Execution

Executing an HIIT session is different from doing regular workouts. In most workouts, you just need to do the workout for a specified period or execute the required the required number of reps. As a result, you may slack off in your execution. When running, some people slow down because they feel lazy. When lifting weights, some people take too much time between reps even when they know that they do not need to rest.

When doing HIIT, these levels of activity are not acceptable. Here are the workout philosophies that you should follow:

Do non-stop workouts

HIIT basically means that you need to do workouts nonstop until the circuit or the routine is over. You do not rest in between workouts. People who do regular workouts usually rest in after doing a set. This is not how you do it with HIIT. If an HIIT circuit lasts for 6 minutes, you should be moving all the time in that period.

Accept the difficulty of the workout

You should take it slow if you are a beginner in working out. You cannot just take an HIIT protocol online and start doing it. Most of the people who post their HIIT workouts are usually of a high level of fitness. A person with no past workout experience will not be able to do the workouts that they suggest.

Instead of trying the workouts suggested by online gurus, you should first try the routines suggested in this book. Most of the workouts here are beginner level exercises. If you find these routines difficult, you may choose to lessen the time per set. If the routine suggests 1 minute of pushups, you may do 30 or 45 seconds instead. This way, you can start doing HIIT and improve your aerobic fitness. You can extend your workout time as you improve your level of fitness.

Work Hard and Fast

The basic idea behind HIIT is to work hard and fast. This is a challenging system but it will show you fast results. For cardio workouts, you only need to run or pedal faster. For strength and calisthenics workouts, you need to do as many reps as you can in the given time without sacrificing your form.

To make sure that you do not slack off or sacrifice your form, you should work out in front of a mirror. By doing it in front of the mirror, you will see signs if you are holding back while working out. You will also see if you are doing movements that make a lift easier. You could then correct your form when you see the mistakes.

There are days when you will feel like you are not in the mood to work hard. In these days, you should review your workouts goals and visualize the body that you want. If it helps, you should also go to the gym that you are familiar with. The presence of other people will encourage you to do your best.

Use workouts that work on large muscle groups

As a beginner, you should work on large muscle groups first when choosing workouts to include in your HIIT routine. These types of workouts usually involve many joints. When you do squats for example, you are moving your knees and your hips. You are also using your core muscles to keep your torso and your spine straight.

Because this type of workout works on many muscle groups in one compound movement, it requires your heart to work harder. By doing these types of workouts, you will make greater improvements in your aerobic fitness.

You should also give special attention to leg workouts when you are choosing what type of exercise you will include in your routines. Some of our largest muscle groups are found in this area. You burn more energy when you use these large muscle groups. Your heart will also work harder because it needs to pump oxygen to these large muscles. In the long run, you will be able to burn more fat if you do a lot of leg workouts.

Don't neglect pre workouts nutrition

HIIT workouts require you to create sudden bursts of energy. Creating these forces with your muscles will use up a lot of your stored energy. Most beginners have not conditioned their bodies to burn stored energy. Their body does not anticipate the intensity of the workout. Because of this, some beginners may experience hypoglycemia in their first few HIIT runs.

To prevent this from happening to you, you should always make sure that you get an adequate pre-workout meal. If your goal is to build muscles, you may also add more protein to your diet through whey protein.

Even if you are not doing any weight lifting sessions in your HIIT, you should still treat it as if you are. You will experience fatigue faster if you do not eat well before an HIIT session.

Adjust your schedule according to how your body feels

We will discuss the 21-day program at the end of the book. In there, we give you instructions on what you should do in each workout day. It is an intensive program to challenge your body. Though the ideal scenario is for all the readers to complete the program, we understand that some people may not be ready for the program yet.

In your case, you should try your best to complete the program. However, if you feel over-fatigue because of doing the workouts, you should take more rest days than suggested.

You should adjust the workouts according to how you feel. The rest and recovery periods are just as important as lifting iron. You should not neglect these rest periods if you want to do HIITs regularly for a long time.

Chapter 2: What Is Hiit?

Just a few short years ago, exercise physiologists believed cardio exercises that raised the heart rate and kept it steady at a moderate rate throughout an entire cardio session was the best form of aerobic exercise for losing weight. They believed that lower-intensity exercise was more effective than high-intensity exercise because the body burned more fat for fuel during extended low-intensity sessions.

As it turns out, they couldn't have been more wrong. HIIT flips that theory on its head, instead opting to have you go all out for brief periods of time, followed by intervals of light to moderate difficulty between the intense sessions.

HIIT is an acronym for **High-Intensity Interval Training**. This relative newcomer to the world of fitness is a form of exercise in which intense sessions of anaerobic exercise are combined with recovery periods consisting of low-intensity exercises to create a training session that is believed to be superior to traditional steady-state aerobic training sessions when it comes to burning fat and building muscle. Additionally, HIIT has been shown to increase cardiovascular ability, improve cholesterol and lower insulin sensitivity.

An example of a simple HIIT session would be 20 minutes worth of intervals of sprinting at full speed for 30 seconds, followed by light jogging for 60 seconds. The 30-second interval is the **high-intensity interval**. It may not seem like much, but is kept short by design, so the exerciser is able to sustain maximum exertion. The 60 seconds of light cardio makes up what is known as the **active recovery interval**, which is time spent engaging in light exercise between the high-intensity intervals in order to allow your body to recharge a bit before the next high-intensity interval begins.

HIIT workouts tend to be shorter than regular workouts, with some of the shortest HIIT workouts clocking in at less than 5 minutes. Don't assume a shorter workout is going to be easier, as newcomers to HIIT often find themselves drenched in sweat and sucking for breath. High-intensity interval training sessions are compact, but there's mounting evidence that appears to prove they're a better choice than steady-state cardio.

While the typical cardio session often ends up feeling like a drawn-out torture session, HIIT offers a more compact workout with sessions of active recovery mixed in. HIIT sessions aren't easy, but a number of exercisers, amateur and professional alike, have found the shorter sessions to be more tolerable than longer cardio sessions.

While most new trends in the world of exercise prove to be nothing more than passing fads, it appears that HIIT is here to stay. HIIT sessions can be designed to fit your individual needs and will produce the results you're looking for quickly. What more could you ask for from a training session?

HIIT Training vs. Interval Training

All high-intensity interval training involves intervals, but not all interval training qualifies as HIIT. There are a lot of people who are engaging in interval training and are calling it HIIT, but aren't actually doing HIIT. I hear guys at the gym all the time claiming to be doing hour-long HIIT routines. When I watch what they're doing, I find they're doing interval training, but it falls short of being actual HIIT.

Interval training involves switching back and forth between different intensities of intervals in a single training session. HIIT does the same thing, but steps it up to the next level by switching between full-intensity intervals and moderate-intensity intervals. If you aren't giving 100% of what you're capable of on every high-intensity interval, you aren't doing HIIT.

Most exercisers aren't capable of giving everything they've got for more than about 30 seconds. A minute of maximum-intensity effort will drain all but the most elite of athletes. The active recovery periods are designed to allow the exerciser just enough time to recover from the maximum-intensity interval to do it again.

Interval training is effective in its own right, but HIIT seeks to step intervals up to a whole new level. HIIT workouts are short by design, usually clocking in at less than 30 minutes (including warm-up and cool-down periods), because most people aren't able to sustain the high level of effort required during HIIT intervals for more than about 20 minutes. If you are able to make it past the 30-minute mark with your intervals, it's probably because you aren't giving it everything you have during the high-intensity interval portions of your routine.

Remember this when determining whether your workout qualifies as a HIIT routine. If you've still got anything left in the gas tank at the end of the workout, it probably wasn't HIIT. High-intensity interval training demands that you put it all on the line. If you still have something left to give, you may not have HIIT it hard enough.

The Many Benefits of HIIT

In addition to weight loss, the following health benefits are believed to be attributed to HIIT:

Boosted metabolism.

Effective fat burning.

Endurance gains.

Improved insulin resistance.

Improvements in cardiovascular health.

Improvements in oxygen uptake.

Reduced muscle loss.

Lower blood pressure.

As you can see, there are a number of benefits associated with HIIT. It's considered one of the best ways to torch fat and it does so in a compact workout that takes up 30 minutes of your day or less.

The Science behind HIIT

While HIIT is currently trending in the world of fitness, there's a decent amount of scientific evidence that appears to back up the claim that shorter bursts of intense exercise are superior to longer sessions of moderate cardio. A number of recent studies have produced results that show HIIT to be an effective means of losing weight, trimming inches off the waistline and improving overall health.

A study published in the Metabolism journal in 1994 compared the effect of both HIIT and endurance training on body fat and skeletal muscle metabolism in healthy young adults. The participants in the study were subjected to either a 15-week HIIT program or a longer 20-week endurance training program. The estimated energy expended by participants in the endurance training program was roughly double that of the participants in the HIIT program, but they didn't see anywhere near double the results. In fact, when adjusted to account for the difference in energy expenditure, the participants in the HIIT program lost more than triple the body fat than those in the steady-state exercise group (1).

Sprint interval training (SIT), which will be covered in-depth in a later chapter, is a form of HIIT in which full-speed sprints are combined with either rest or active recovery periods.

A 2010 study looked at the effect of SIT training on overweight and obese men and found that participants who completed a 2-week SIT intervention consisting of 30-second sprints followed by 4 ½ minute rest periods showed a significant reduction in both waist and hip circumference. Oxygen uptake and insulin sensitivity showed marked improvement after sprint interval training and systolic blood pressure was lower for at least 24 hours post-intervention. This effect was short-lived, as blood pressure, insulin sensitivity and oxygen uptake all returned to close to baseline when measurements were taken 72 hours after the intervention (2).

What this appears to indicate is HIIT exercise can help you lose inches off both your waistline and your hips, with the added bonus of potentially lowering blood pressure and improving insulin sensitivity. HIIT may even help you breathe easier and more deeply, but the effects are going to be short-lived if you stop exercising and return to leading a sedentary lifestyle.

A 2005 study looked at the connection between intensity of exercise and its effect on blood lipids. The participants were asked to perform 8 different exercises consisting of 20 repetitions of a light load or 8 exercises of 10 repetitions of a heavier load. They were then asked to wait 7 days, after which they were asked to perform whichever of the sets of exercises they hadn't previously performed. Blood was drawn before, right after and 15 minutes after the last exercise was complete. It was determined that intense exercise increased HDL cholesterol, which is good cholesterol in the body, immediately after high-intensity exercise (3).

These are just a handful of the many studies that seem to indicate HIIT is more than just a passing fad. Here are a few more that appear to tie HIIT to a number of health benefits:

A 2008 University of South Wales study of the effect of HIIT on young women found performing HIIT 3 times a week for 15 weeks produced significant reductions in total body fat while improving insulin resistance when compared to the same amount of steady-state exercise (4).

A study of subjects who cycle regularly found that aerobic power, exercise work rates and peak power output were all increased after interval training (5).

An East Tennessee State University study of obese women found that HIIT improved aerobic power, body composition and resting metabolic rate when compared to low-intensity steady state training (6).

Most of the studies of HIIT have been published in the last 10 years and have produced largely positive results. HIIT appears to be an effective means of lowering body fat while taking inches off of all of the areas that matter. It also appears to be a means through which you can maximize weight loss while minimizing the amount of muscle being lost to atrophy.

Keep a watchful eye on the studies of HIIT currently being done by the scientific community. Since HIIT is a relative newcomer to the world of fitness, it's highly likely that all of the health benefits haven't yet been discovered. There may be additional health benefits of HIIT just waiting to be unlocked.

Marathon Runners vs. Sprinters

In case you need further proof HIIT allows you to lose fat while retaining and possibly even building muscle, let's take a quick look at the difference between marathon runners and Olympic sprinters.

At a glance, you'll immediately notice marathon runners are thin and appear to have little by way of muscle on their bodies. These runners endure long, intense training sessions designed to improve their stamina to the point where they're able to run long distances while maintaining a certain speed. Marathon runners don't run fast. Instead, they run for a long time at a slower speed than the top speed they're capable of. Elite marathon athletes often find themselves running in excess of 100 miles per week, placing them firmly at the extreme end of steady-state athletes.

Extended periods of aerobic exercise isn't conducive to muscle growth, so marathon runners tend to be thin and lanky. To be fair, Olympic marathon runners are in prime condition and are elite athletes who are able to withstand rigorous training regimens; they just don't tend to have much muscle mass on their bodies.

On the other hand, an Olympic sprinter is more often than not a sight to behold. Olympic sprinters have bulging muscles and have significantly more muscle mass than marathon runners. Sprinters train every bit as hard as marathon runners, but they don't train for endurance. They train for short bursts of intense speed because they aren't in their races for the long haul. They're looking to win a short race run at the fastest speeds humanly possible. In short, they fall at the extreme end of high-intensity training.

While nobody would make the argument that marathon runners are out of shape, I would argue that I'd rather look like a sprinter than a marathon runner when it's all said and done. Not that looking like a marathon runner is a bad thing; I'd just rather have all my hard work pay off in added muscle mass combined with fat loss instead of fat loss at the expense of muscle mass.

Short, fast bursts of intense cardio exercise will help you to lose fat without robbing your body of muscle size and fullness. If there's any doubt, look up pictures of marathon runners and sprinters on your computer and compare them side-by-side.

HIIT Burns More Calories

The intensity and duration of HIIT intervals allows you to really step up the pace of your workout, which results in your body burning a larger number of calories in a shorter amount of time. A good HIIT routine can burn more calories in 20 minutes of work than most people burn in an hour of steady-state cardio.

The real benefit of HIIT lies in something known amongst HIIT enthusiasts as the "**afterburn**." This is the effect HIIT has on the body after the workout, as the body continues to burn calories well after the workout is complete in an attempt to restore itself back to a resting state. This afterburn effect is believed to last for a day or two after an intense HIIT workout. This effect is practically non-existent when it comes to steady-state cardio.

It's recommended you space your HIIT workouts out with a day or two between them in order to take full advantage of afterburn effect. Your body hasn't fully recovered a day later and you'll be placing additional stress on it by working out too soon.

Chapter 3: What Is High-Intensity Interval Training?

Looking young and beautiful, as well as being fit, doesn't just happen through eating right, though a big chunk of it is reliant on correct diet. But equally important is getting enough physical training in, especially when talking about being fit, in which case, you'll need to pair correct eating with getting regular exercise.

But not all exercises are created equal and an exercise or workout program by any other name won't work as good as high-intensity interval training. Different types of exercises are superior over others depending on your goal. If your goal is to achieve excellent cardiovascular fitness, then simply brisk walking or going for regular runs in the morning are the optimal workouts for such a goal. If your goal is to get muscularly huge just like

Dwayne "The Rock" Johnson, you'll need to get into a seriously heavy weight-lifting program. But if your goal is to achieve a lean body that looks beautifully fit – for the ladies – or muscularly ripped but not huge like the body of Zac Efron, then High-Intensity Interval Training may just be what the physical fitness doctor ordered.

So, what is High-Intensity Interval Training – or HIIT for short? Basically, it's an exercise program that involves alternating high-intensity exercises with either a short period of rest or low-intensity exercises. A good example of this would be running as fast as you can for 20 seconds then brisk walking for another 20 seconds before repeating the cycle several times over. People who've done HIIT will attest to the fact that a HIIT program – most of which are bodyweight exercises – done for even just 20 minutes is so much more effective in terms of burning calories compared to brisk walking for about an hour.

HIIT Phases

Physiologically speaking, it's downright impossible to sustain maximum physical effort during exercise over an extended period of time. The main reason for this is because human bodies weren't wired to use calories in such a way. To give you a better idea of how your body burns calories during exercise, let's say that you run outdoors – at the fastest speed, you can run – for 20 minutes. Here's what happens to your body, a.k.a., the HIIT phases.

- The Phosphocreatine Phase: During the first 20 seconds or less of your sprint, things are pretty much okay – excellent! You feel like a Ferrari speeding down the Autobahn even if you're more like fixed-gear bike speeding down the streets of

New York. You're Usain Bolt trapped in a mortal's body. Life's good! You know why? It's because, at the earliest phase of your sprint, your body is utilizing its phosphocreatine stores, which is a source of high-intensity energy.

• Anaerobic Glycolysis Phase: After the first 20 seconds or so, your body will have spent much of its phosphocreatine stores, at which point your body will shift to the Anaerobic Glycolysis phase, wherein your body will use more lactic acid than phosphocreatine as its main source of fuel. At this point, you'll feel like you're still exerting max effort but your running speed will have significantly reduced. You'll also start feeling like your lungs are working very, very hard.

Unless you're an elite athlete at the levels of Usain Bolt or LeBron James, the chances of you being able to sustain this for even just 10 minutes are very, very low. If your physical conditioning is below average or even just average, you'd probably have to slow down or worse, stop running altogether. And if you have been a couch potato for a long time, it's highly possible that you might even puke, which is a normal occurrence for sedentary people who do this for the first time, as a result of the sudden change in blood acidity levels (remember lactic acid?).

When you break everything down to the level of laymen's terms, the reason why it's impossible to exert maximum effort beyond a short window of time can be summed up in one word.

Oxygen

Yep, that's it. It's the magical molecule. In particular, it's all about demand and supply during maximum exertion of effort. During high-intensity effort, demand for oxygen skyrockets to levels that are much more than the body can provide. It's basically a choice between efficiency and intensity, i.e., the higher the intensity the lower the efficiency and vice versa.

If you work out with low intensity, like when you're just walking around the mall, the primary process by which your body utilizes energy is called aerobic metabolism. What does this mean? To break down fat and carbohydrates for fuel, your body needs oxygen. But while this process is great for efficiency, e.g., the ability to sustain an action for longer periods of time like running marathons, it sucks for activities that require intensity such as all-out sprints.

When you're exerting maximum or near maximum effort (high-intensity activities), anaerobic metabolism takes over. What does this mean? As mentioned earlier, high-intensity exercises tend to demand oxygen at levels that far exceed your body's ability to provide it where needed. In a state of anaerobic metabolism, your body compensates for the lack of oxygen by releasing short bursts of high energy or speed.

Given these 2 seemingly opposite metabolic processes, is it possible to get the best of both worlds, especially for getting fit and looking young and fab? This is where HIIT comes into play!

With high-intensity interval training, you will alternate anaerobic with aerobic metabolism, i.e., alternate short bursts of high-intensity activities with relatively long periods of low-intensity exercises like walking or complete rest. During the short bursts of high-intensity exercises, you'll be able to promote a huge metabolic demand that can be very powerful in terms of burning off body fat, and achieving much greater fitness and conditioning levels. And during the low or no intensity periods, you allow your body to shift to the aerobic energy system and recover appropriately so you can give those short high-intensity bursts several more goes.

Hormones

Another important component of HIIT is hormones. Stress hormones are very low in low to no intensity exercises like tai chi or yoga. Under normal circumstances, low-stress hormone levels are great for the body. But for optimal fat loss and fitness, you'll need to substantially up the ante even for just a short period of time.

When you do HIIT, your oxygen consumption or demand may reach up to 90% of your VO2max, which is a primary measure of cardiovascular fitness and effort. At this level, your body produces much higher levels of key stress hormones such as aldosterone, cortisol, norepinephrine (noradrenaline) and epinephrine (or adrenaline). As a response to these elevated levels, your body triggers higher production of growth hormones and testosterone, both of which are very important for burning fat, gaining muscle mass, and achieving optimum fitness. Taken together, all these hormones have the power to substantially alter your body's anabolism and composition.

Important HIIT Stuff

Because HIIT workouts are – as the name implies – intense by nature, they can significantly raise your stress hormones. Doing HIIT workouts – as with most high-intensity physical activities – can put your body in what's called as a "crisis" state, i.e., oxygen delivery to tissues are compromised, body temperature rises, fuel stores and body fluids are significantly depleted, and this can lead to tissue damage. Consequently, your body reacts defensively to such a state by producing endocrine, which is similar to what psychological stresses, physical injuries, low blood sugar levels, dehydration, elevated body temperature, acidosis, elevated carbon dioxide levels, and low blood oxygen levels can do to the body.

To put it simply, your body starts to freak out at this stage. When it does, it will tend to bring out its "nuclear weapons" it's i.e., its primary defensive weapons. HIIT and other high-intensity physical activities can put so much stress on your body, forcing it to eventually adapt as a survival mechanism.

Why Bother With HIIT?

Despite HIIT subjecting your body to huge amounts of stress, albeit for short periods only, performing this type of workout can give you several significant benefits:

- Accelerated fat loss while sparing muscle mass;

- Substantial improvement in cardiovascular health and fitness;

- Much improved sport-centric energy systems;

- Ability to perform high-intensity activities for longer periods of time;

- Improved resiliency, perseverance, and tolerance of discomfort, i.e., a much tougher mind; and

- Increased activation of fast-twitch muscles, which are important for optimal fitness, power, and strength.

Even better, all these benefits can be enjoyed through much shorter workout times. For example, a mere 5 to 10 minutes of HIIT can help you burn more calories than a 30-minute jog or an hour of brisk walking. Can you imagine that? More for less!

How to HIIT Your Way to Fitness, Strength, Youth and Beauty

You can perform HIIT workouts in practically an infinite number of ways using a myriad number of exercise combos. But despite the huge number of possible ways to do HIIT, all you need to remember is its basic principle: alternating short periods of high-intensity exercises with low-intensity work or rest/recovery. It's that simple!

Many studies have already been conducted on HIIT but one of the most meaningful ones is called The Tabata

Study, where the study's participants were asked to row for intervals, i.e., they were asked to row at an ultra-fast pace for 20 seconds followed by a 10-second recovery of relaxed rowing and repeat the cycle 8 times for a total time of 4 minutes. The participants registered a remarkable 28% jump in an average anaerobic capacity as well as a 14% jump in average VO2max.

It's from the study's methodology that the Tabata protocol for HIIT came about. In particular, the protocol requires alternating 20 seconds of high-intensity work with 10 seconds of low intensity or rest periods, which was the pattern used during the study itself. The Tabata protocol is probably the most popular HIIT protocol today.

Resistance Exercises and HIIT

One of the best ways to optimize your HIIT workouts is by performing resistance exercises, i.e., weights. You can use either your own bodyweight or barbells and dumbbells for HIIT. In particular, the best resistance exercises for HIIT are compound or multi-joint exercises, which use more than 1 single body part to perform like pushups, pull ups and the like. Collectively, such exercises are called "oxygen vampires" by some people in the business.

If at some point your body has already started to adapt to the stress of specific exercises, you can "re-stress" your body by combining it with others to up the ante. Many of the exercises I'll show you later are combos, which can really make your lungs and muscles feel like they're gonna blow!

Personalized HIITs

The beautiful thing with HIIT is that with its very simple principle of alternating high- intensity exercises with low-intensity ones or rest, it can be very easy for you to create your own personalized HIIT workout programs. Just like your wardrobe, you can mix and match different exercises while utilizing HIIT. You don't need to be a certified trainer to create your own workouts in the long run.

Another benefit of the customizability of HIIT is that you can lower your risks for injuries. How? By being able to easily mix things up, you can minimize your risks for overtraining, which is one of the leading causes of exercise-related injuries. By mixing and matching, you also minimize what's possibly your biggest risk ever – boredom.

More than just mixing and matching specific exercises, you can also change the duration of your intervals. While the Tabata protocol is a very effective one for most people, it doesn't mean it's your only option. Keep in mind that everybody has their own unique circumstances and characteristics and it's possible that a longer or shorter high-intensity duration may work better for you, which can last anywhere from 10 to 60 seconds.

You can also work with maintaining the high-intensity duration but increasing that of the low intensity or rest intervals for optimum recovery. These can be anywhere from 10 seconds to more than a minute. Don't be afraid to experiment and discover what's optimal for your body.

If you're a complete beginner to exercise – or even with HIIT only – it's best to err on the side of caution by keeping high-intensity intervals short and rest or low-intensity intervals longer. As you get a feel of how your body responds to HIIT, you can adjust accordingly.

Intensity Levels

Many beginners make a mistake of assuming that intensity is generic, i.e., what's high intensity for one is the same for another person. Don't make the same mistake. Intensity levels are relative to the person performing the exercise him or herself. And while there are very accurate but complicated methods for determining exercise intensity, you have a relatively accurate and practical way of determining whether or not you're performing exercises or intervals at a high intensity: the talk test.

Here's how the talk test goes. Try talking as if you're engaged in a conversation with someone while performing your exercises. If you're able to talk with very little effort or difficulty, as if you're having a nice conversation with a friend in a coffee shop, that's low intensity. If you're able to talk but with a slight effort to breathe and talk normally, that's mid intensity. If you can barely talk – now that's high intensity!

Easy, isn't it?

Now suppose you find yourself performing at less than high intensity – how can you up the ante use the same exercises? One way is to increase the speed by which you perform the exercise. If you're able to do, say 10 pushups in 15 seconds, increase it to 13 pushups in 15 seconds.

If you're using barbells or dumbbells at the gym, you can also increase the weight you're lifting. If you're using bodyweight exercises, which is what all of the 100 exercises I'll be teaching you, later on, are so you have no reason not to do HIIT anywhere you are, you can change your body's angle or elevation instead.

Warming Up and Cooling Down

When exercising, especially if it's high intensity, warm-ups are crucial to minimizing the risk of any injuries like torn ligaments, pulled muscles or lightheadedness due to an abrupt start. When it comes to warming and limbering up the muscles, there are two types of stretches: dynamic and static. Dynamic stretches involve movement, examples of which include brisk walking, bodyweight squats, jogging and arm circles, among others. These are best for warming and limbering up because it allows your muscles to loosen up gradually through repetitive actions. Static stretches, on the other hand, aren't as beneficial for starting your HIIT workouts because this forces your muscles to stretch as far as they can without the benefit of limbering or warming up first. It's like going from 0 to 150 mph in 10 seconds! Static stretches include, among others, chest stretches, hamstring stretches and thigh stretches, among others and are best for cooling down, i.e., post workout.

Chapter 4: Types Of Hiit

Through the years, different regimens following the basic HIIT principle have been developed by various fitness experts. Here are some of them:

Peter Coe Regimen. One type of HIIT was used in the 1970s by coach Peter Coe. This was an exercise with noticeably short recovery phases. The regimen was originally designed by the coach for his son Sebastian Cole, an Olympic Gold Medalist. This system was inspired by the principles of German university professor and coach Woldemar Gerschler and Swedish Physiologist Per-Olof Astrand. The sessions consisted of repeated full-intensity 200-meter runs, with only half a minute of recovery between each run.

Tabata Regimen. A more well-known regimen, the Tabata was based on a 1996 study conducted by Japanese professor Izumi Tabata and his colleagues. The study originally done involving Olympic speed skaters. They were made to exercise intensely for 20-seconds (by intense, here we mean almost double their normal maximal aerobic capacity - think almost twice the limit of your lungs). Then, they were followed up with 10 seconds of rest. This is repeated continuously for four minutes or eight cycles. It was initially called the IE1 protocol, and performed on cycle ergometer that is mechanically braked.

During the course of the original study, the athletes have used this method to train four times a week. The fifth day was spent in steady-state training. The gain obtained was actually similar to those reached by athletes on a steady-state regimen five times a week! The HIIT group also had an overall greater gain, since they started with a lower aerobic efficiency. They were the only group that gained benefits in the field of anaerobic capacity. This is a simple illustration of our point earlier: the greater the after burn, the greater the benefits.

Gibala Regimen. In Canada's McMaster University, Professor Martin Gibala has been conducting researches on the nature of high-intensity workouts for several years. Last 2009, they did a study on students who used 3 minutes of warm-up time, 60 seconds of intense workouts at near maximum capacity, and 75 seconds of rest to cap. This is repeated over 8-12 cycles. This process has sometimes been referred to as the "Little Method".

Despite the demeaning name, the subjects used this method to train 3 times a week and overall gained benefits that would be similar to those had by others who trained with steady-state routines at a little more than half of full capacity, five times a week. Even as it is more demanding than most regimens, the Little Method compensated by being available to the public using nothing more complex than an exercise bike.

In 2011, a less intense version was published by Gibala's group in the paper "Medicine & Science in Sports & Exercise". The alternative was supposed to be a friendlier alternative for people who have not had any regular form of exercise in more than a year. This system used the same 3 minutes of warm-up exercises, followed by 10 reps of 60-second workouts at more than half the exerciser's limits, alternating with a minute of rest in between each repetition. After these is a 5-minute cool-down exercise.

Timmons Regimen. At the University of Loughborough in Leicestershire, systems biology professor Jamie Timmons advocates the use of a few short exercise bursts, conducted at complete intensity. This was tested by none other than BBC Journalist Michael Mosley during a 2012 documentary program. Professor Timmons utilizes a biking regimen of three sets.

Each set consists of 2 minutes of gentle bike work, alternating with 20-second bursts at maximum intensity. This is to be done three times a week, with around three minutes of full-intensity exercises every week. Some warm up and recovery time is also to be factored in.

One of the more profound effects of this exercise is its ability to improve some aspects of a person's health, including the increased sensitivity to insulin that was discussed earlier.

Chapter 5: Weekly Trainings To Get Stronger, Faster, Lighter

The HIIT cycling program that will be discussed in the following chapter will be divided into three stages; the beginner, intermediate, and expert stages. For best results, you need to choose the stage that is appropriate for your level of fitness.

The beginner stage

This stage is perfect for people who have been living a sedentary lifestyle prior to the HIIT program. It is focused on improving your cardiovascular health to prepare you for the next stages of the program. Just like in any beginner workout program, the beginner stage of the High Intensity Interval Cycling Training will have a long warm-up period. It also has longer durations for the low intensity part of the training.

After the beginner stage, you will have muscles that are ready for the later stages. The muscles that have weakened because of the sedentary lifestyle will become ready for more rigorous types of workout tasks. In this stage, there will already be a short duration of high intensity biking. These short sprints will activate your fast twitch muscles. This type of muscles fibers is the least used by people who are living a sedentary lifestyle. People who are not accustomed to sprinting often expose these muscles to injury when they instantly expose them to high intensity workouts. Through this stage, you will allow them to start working with the minimal risk of injury. The long warm-up periods will also allow this type of muscles to heat up and become more flexible before they are exposed to sprinting.

You should also take into consideration that you will be experiencing some muscle pains due to the lactic acid accumulation in the muscles. This may happen after sprinting and may linger on after the workout. This type of pain may be paralyzing at first but as you become more familiar with the sensation, you will become desensitized from it. Many bikers experience the same thing and they have developed a tolerance to the pain caused by the process. Your aim is to develop the same type of tolerance in your beginner stage.

This stage is also designed to make you feel comfortable with breathing while you are on the bike. Breathing is the key to longer performances. In the beginning, you will struggle to catch your breath after sprints. As you become more experienced, your breathing will be able to transition between sprints and low intensity speeds smoothly.

Breathing is most important during the low intensity phase of the workout. This is the time for aerobic respiration. At this phase, you should keep your mind focused in your breathing. People who take their breathing for granted in this stage often take shallow breaths resulting to a lack of oxygen in their inhalation. Their body will try to compensate for the lack of oxygen by breathing faster. The fast breathing combined with inadequate supply of oxygen will cause them to tire faster.

For a longer performance, you should practice doing deep regular breathing. During aerobic respiration, your body will be producing a lot carbon dioxide. Deep exhalation allows your body to release the carbon dioxide faster. Deep breathing during the low intensity phase of the workout also prevents the body from relying on anaerobic respiration. This will lessen the amount of lactic acid accumulation in your muscles.

You will only do this workout 3x a week. This will give you more time to do other types of workouts on the other days of the week. It will also give your thigh and calf muscles time to heal for the next HIIT biking session. The 3-day weekly workout will increase the rate of your metabolism. Exercise naturally increases that but it begins to slow down again 24 hours after working out. By working out every other day, your metabolism will have no time to slow down. Maintaining a fast metabolic rate will help you burn more fats when you are in your rested state.

Day of the week	HIIT Program

Monday	Warm up for 8 minutes: Your normal biking pace
	Resistance: Low
	Rest: 2 minutes
	Workout:
	10 seconds high intensity (sprints), 1 minute low intensity (repeat 6 times)
	Rest: 1 minute

	10 seconds high intensity (sprints), 1 minute low intensity (repeat 6 times)
	Total workout time: 25 minutes
Tuesday	Strength training day
Wednesday	Warm up for 8 minutes: Your normal biking pace

Resistance: Low

Rest: 2 minutes

Workout:

10 seconds high intensity (sprints), 1 minute low intensity (repeat 6 times)

Rest: 1 minute

10 seconds high intensity (sprints), 1 minute low

	intensity (repeat 6 times)
	Total workout time: 25 minutes
Thursday	Strength training day
Friday	Warm up for 8 minutes: Your normal biking pace
	Resistance: Low
	Rest: 2 minutes

Workout:

15 seconds high intensity (sprints), 1 minute low intensity (repeat 6 times)

Rest: 1 minute

15 seconds high intensity (sprints), 1 minute low intensity (repeat 6 times)

Total workout time:

	25 minutes
Saturday	Strength training day
Sunday	Rest day

You should do this workout routine for one month. Unlike regular endurance training, HIIT routines don't need 45 minutes to burn fats. You need to focus more on improving the power in your sprints and keeping your breathing regular.

After one month, you could now try the workout routine of the intermediate stage. If you become out of breath while doing it, you can spend some more time using the beginner stage routine until your endurance has developed for the next level.

Intermediate stage

You can start with the intermediate stage after your first month. In this stage, the intensity of the workout will begin to increase. There will be shorter warm-up and rest periods. In the previous stage, the high intensity-low intensity ratio was 10 seconds is to 1 minute or 1:6. On the Friday sessions, we increased it to 15 seconds is to 1 minute or 1:4. In this stage we will bring them closer and make the workout a bit more challenging.

At the end of this stage, your calf and thigh muscles will significantly improve. These muscles will become more accustomed to generating busts of energy. You will be more accustomed to sprinting and your tolerance towards the pain caused by the lactic acid will also increase.

The longer duration of the workout sessions will also significantly increase your cardio-respiratory resistance. Combined with the proper deep breathing method during the low intensity phase of the workout, you will be able to last longer during workouts. Improving your resistance for long rides will prepare your body for the time when you will start working out on the road.

In this stage, we will also introduce the super set. A super set is a workout session that is longer than your usual duration. You do this when you still feel like working out even after your usual routine is done. It could also include a closer high intensity-low intensity ratio.

The HIIT superset will help you burn fat much faster. After the first 20 minutes of workout, your body will begin tapping into your energy reserves. This is the reason behind your fat loss. Most of the time, the fat loss will come from your tummy or your chest. Using a super set will prolong the duration that your body is using your fat reserves. This will result to more fat loss per session when compared to your regular workout.

Because the duration and the intensity of the workout in a HIIT superset are increased, you may need more time to recover from it. In our Monday-Wednesday-Friday workout schedule, the best time to do it is on Friday. This will give your calf and thigh muscles more time to recover before the next HIIT bike session.

Day of the week	HIIT Program
Monday	Warm up for 5

minutes: Your normal biking pace

Resistance: Low

Rest: 1 minutes

Workout:

30 seconds high intensity (sprints), 1 minute low intensity (repeat 8 times)

Rest: 1 minute

	30 seconds high intensity (sprints), 1 minute low intensity (repeat 5 times)
	Total workout time: 26 minutes and 30 seconds
Tuesday	Strength training day
Wednesday	Warm up for 5 minutes: Your normal biking pace

Resistance: Low

Rest: 1 minutes

Workout:

30 seconds high intensity (sprints), 1 minute low intensity (repeat 8 times)

Rest: 1 minute

30 seconds high intensity (sprints), 1 minute low

	intensity (repeat 5 times)
	Total workout time: 26 minutes and 30 seconds
Thursday	Strength training day
Friday	Warm up for 5 minutes: Your normal biking pace
	Resistance: Low
	Rest: 1 minutes

Workout:

30 seconds high intensity (sprints), 1 minute low intensity (repeat 8 times)

Rest: 1 minute

40 seconds high intensity (sprints), 1 minute low intensity (repeat 5 times)

Total workout time:

	27 minutes
Saturday	Strength training day
Sunday	Rest day
Superset Day	Warm up for 10 minutes: Your normal biking pace
	Resistance: Medium
	Rest: 1 minutes

Workout:

Resistance: Low

30 seconds high intensity (sprints), 1 minute low intensity (repeat 5 times)

Rest: 1 minute

30 seconds high intensity (sprints), 1 minute low intensity (repeat 5 times)

Rest: 1 minute

40 seconds high intensity (sprints), 1 minute low intensity (repeat 3 times)

Total workout time: 33 minutes

If you don't have a lot of experience being on a bike, you should stay on the intermediate stage for at least 2 months. You should try to narrow down the high intensity-low intensity ratio to make the routine more challenging.

If you are in a country with a hot climate, you will sweat a lot especially when doing a super set. You should have energy bars and energy drinks ready in case of dehydration and hypoglycemia.

Expert stage

Before you move on to the expert, you should make sure that you are ready for long distance biking because this is the stage where you will go out on the road. When you are on the road, you should remember to reserve some energy for the trip back. Start with small distance rides and increase your distance on each trip.

You should also know the basics of going on a cycling trip. You should plan out your route to get back home on time. Sprinting on your bike is not a good idea in the busy city streets. You should make sure that the route you take will be free of heavy traffic and pedestrians. If you have bike lanes in your city streets, you should focus your route on those lanes.

The expert stage is a combination of stationary bike and road workouts. The amount of road workout that you do depends on how much time you can devote to it. If you are a weekend warrior, you should plan your weekend around your road biking sessions.

In this stage, you should follow the routine of the intermediate stage. You should then add a superset after the day's routine. You should try to finish the superset or push until you are out of air.

Day of the week	HIIT Program	

Monday	Intermediate Stage Routine
	Super Set
Tuesday	Strength training day
Wednesday	Intermediate Stage Routine
	Super Set
Thursday	Strength training day
Friday	Intermediate Stage Routine
	Super Set

Saturday	Strength training day
Sunday	Rest day
Superset Day	Warm up for 10 minutes: Your normal biking pace
	Resistance: Medium
	Rest: 1 minutes
	Workout:
	Resistance: Low

30 seconds high intensity (sprints), 1 minute low intensity (repeat 5 times)

Rest: 1 minute

30 seconds high intensity (sprints), 1 minute low intensity (repeat 5 times)

Rest: 1 minute

40 seconds high intensity (sprints), 1 minute low intensity (repeat 3 times)

	Total workout time: 33 minutes

On the road, you should find the best leg in your route where you can sprint. Use the intermediate stage routine while travelling in this part of the route. You should avoid places however, that have a lot of sharp turns. You should also avoid doing HIIT routines on areas that have a lot of cliffs. Highways in plains outside of the urban areas are the best type of road to use your bike in.

Chapter 6: Hiit Workouts For The Home

Sometimes, we just don't have the time to go to the gym or go for that long run around the park and that is where HIIT steps in. You don't need loads of equipment and you don't need loads of time to get the benefits. For the workouts below, all you need is kettlebells, dumbbells of a medicine ball at the absolute most. Some of the exercises will only require your own bodyweight, nothing else, and all can be done in the comfort of your own home.

Ready? Then let's begin!

For all of these workouts, please warm up for a period of three to five minutes using jumping jacks, running on the spot or skipping with a rope. This is important – HIIT is intensive exercise and if you don't warm your muscles up, you are running a very high risk of injury.

Exercise Directions

Exercises one through four:

Although these contain resistance training you can still do them for HIIT. Each exercise should be done for one minute with weights that are light enough to ensure that you keep the proper form. You are going to go through these four very quickly so make your weight lighter than one you would use for strength training.

Between each one, do 30 seconds of jump squats or mountain climbers and rest for 15 seconds or less. After each round (exercises one through four with all the other bits) rest up for three minutes and the then repeat twice more.

Exercise 1

Kettlebell Swings

Bend the knees so they are at an angle of 90 degrees. Your feet should be just over shoulder-width apart, your back should be leaning forward slightly and you should have a kettle bell held between your legs. Start your swing upwards, thrusting the hips forward and bring the kettlebell up to your shoulder height. Return to your starting position

Decline Pushups

Put your hands flat on the floor with your head facing down and both of your feet onto a bench. Make sure your back is straight and then lower your body down until your elbows are at a 90-degree angle and the humorous bone is parallel to the floor. Return and repeat

Fire Hydrants

Start off on all fours. Your hands should be about shoulder-width apart, your head facing down, your back straight. Use your hip abductor to raise one leg to the side, until it is parallel to the floor. Return and repeat with the other leg.

Exercise 2

Forward Dumbbell Lunge with a Twist

Stand up straight and hold a dumbbell out to the front of you. Step forward into a lunge keeping your knees level with or behind your toes and your back knee must not be on the ground. Twist slowly to one side keeping the dumbbell held out in front. Return to the center and push off to your start position. Repeat on the other side

Bent Lateral Raise using Dumbbells

Lean forward but keep your back straight and hold out a dumbbell in each hand, straight in front of you but below knee level. Raise the dumbbells up slowly until they are level to your shoulders, but still keeping a straight back and with your head looking down. Lower the dumbbells back to the start position and repeat.

Plank with a Dumbbell Row

Get into position for a push-up, with your feet apart shoulder-width, your head looking down and your back straight. You will be holding a pair of dumbbells. Retaining your position, lift with one dumbbell towards your abdominal muscles and hold it for one second. Drop your arm back to the starting position slowly and repeat with the other.

Exercise 3

Weighted Step-ups

Begin by holding a dumbbell in each hand and put one foot up on a bench. Lift up your body off the ground, generating the power using the leg on the bench. When you reach the top, switch over to the other food and go back down. Repeat for the opposite side.

Chin-ups

Use an underhand grip to hold a bar with our hands shoulder-width apart. Your knees should be at a 90-degree angle. Lift your body slowly until your chin is over the bar; return to start and repeat

Russian Twists

Lie on the floor, bending your knees to a 90-degree angle and your heels on the floor. Hold out a medicine ball to the front of you with your arms straight and twist from side to side, keeping your back at an angle.

Exercise 4

Weighted Goblet Squats

Holding a kettle bell with both of your hands, bring it up under your chin. Twist your feet so your toes are turned out at an angle of 30 degrees. Now go into a squat, making sure your knees push out and your elbows move between your knees. Take it as low as you possibly can while retaining your back arch and then return slowly to your start position

Decline Pushups – see above

Plank with a Dumbbell Row – see above

Exercises five through eight:

Perform between 15 and 20 repetitions of each exercise with a 10 second or less break in between each exercise. Repeat until you have worked out for 10 minutes.

Exercise 5:

Wall Squat and Pulse on the Toes

Start with your back flat to the wall and then slide down until you are at a 90-degree angle at the waist and knees. Now press back up through the balls of the toes, bringing your calf muscles into play. Slide up and down the wall continuously for three to five inches for 15 seconds.

Rest for five seconds by returning to a standing position and then lowering down slowly.

Power Pushup and Mountain Climbers

This is similar to a normal push up but instead, you don't just straighten the arms, you push up off the ground, using all your strength and your power and land on your elbows softly. Then do 10 mountain climbers – push your knees to your chest five times on each knee and make them as explosive as you can while retaining form.

A Walking Plank

Begin in the plank position resting your forearms flat on the ground. Now walk up into a full plank – put your palms flat on the ground and straighten your elbows out. Return to the forearm plank. Make sure you stay steady and controlled at all times and keep your butt and hips in line with your body and engage your abs.

Exercise 6:

Tuck Jumps

Begin in a squat position with your chest up and your knees tucked behind your toes. Now jump, go as high as you possibly can and push your knees into your chest. Land with soft knees on the balls of your feet and lower your heels down. Be quick and intense with this and try not to have a break in between the jumps

Woodchoppers

You can use a big bottle of washing detergent for this, the heavier the better. Begin with your feet flat on the floor, hip-width distance and your knees should be bent in a half-squat. Turn your body one way to the outer edge of your foot. Tighten up your abdominals and swing your body and your arms holding the detergent, up to the opposite corner, just like you were swinging a golf club. Make sure your feet stay flat to the floor at all times and repeat equally on both sides.

Bear Crawl and Reverse Burpee

Get into squat position and then walk your hands to a plank position. Now do a reverse burpee – push your knees to your chest, jump up straight and land in a squat. Your legs shoot back to a plank position and then do a single pushup. Now walk the hands back to the feet and go back to your start position. Keep your movements smooth

Exercise 7:

Mountain Climbers

For this, you need two towels. Start in a plank position and have each foot on a towel. Bring your knees up to your chest twice on each side for a total of four and then push your knee outwards to your elbow twice on each side.

Squat Jump and Overhead Press

Get yourself a gallon bottle of water – this will weigh about 8.5 lbs. Hold it at chest, keeping your feet together and your elbows in. Jump your legs to just over hip-width and go straight to a full squat, holding the water above you. Now jump your feet back together and bring the water back down to your chest. Do this as quickly as you can.

Walking Plank – see above

Exercise 8:

Knee Tucks

Use a towel and do this on a slippery surface. Put the towel beneath your feet and begin in a plank position. Push your knees to your chest while sliding the feet forward but keeping your butt down.

High Knees and Squat Jumps

Keep your back straight and push your knees to your chest, just as though you were running up the stairs. Land on the balls of the feet with soft knees. Do five on each side and follow this with three jump squats – begin in a squat position with your chest up and your knees tucked behind your toes and your weight on your heels. Jump up as far as you can and return to a squat, ensuring your knees bend when you land.

Bear Crawl and Reverse Burpee – see above

Exercise 9:

Do these next two movements like this:

10 push-ups

A cross body mountain climber – a left and a right = 1

9 push-ups

2 cross body mountain climbers

8 push-ups

3 cross body mountain climbers

Continue till you get to one pushup and 20 of the mountain climbers

Exercise 10:

Do a Tabata workout of 12 minutes with 20 seconds of intense work and 10 seconds of rest

Cycle through the following eight times:

Squats – 20 seconds

Rest – 10 seconds

Burpees – 20 seconds

Rest – 10 seconds

Sit-ups – 20 seconds

Rest – 10 seconds

Chapter 7: Hiit Myths

HIIT appears to be the perfect solution for weight loss, muscle gain and improved stamina. However, with all the good and bad claims relating to high intensity training, it can be confusing. Below are the common myths associated with HIIT:

1. HIIT should be done daily

HIIT should only be done twice or three times a week, to allow your muscles to rest and regenerate. Daily intense workouts are not practical, as it requires a high level of energy and concentration, which people don't normally have. Also, HIIT causes muscle pain after the workout and it takes one to two days for the body to recover.

HIIT is beneficial for people who don't abuse their body and workout program.

You need to read your own body and adjust accordingly to avoid overtraining and associated injuries.

2. HIIT is limited to sprinting and sprinters

HIIT can be done indoors or outdoors. It is also not limited to sprinting or jogging alone. Though sprinting is commonly used in many HIIT programs, there are a lot of other exercises being used too. These are, jumping jacks, high knees, mountain climbers, burpees, and walking to name a few.

It is not only beneficial for sprinters, but for athletes or people who want to increase their stamina and increase metabolism.

3. HIIT follows strict eating patterns

HIIT does not follow a scheduled eating plan. There are no required pre or post intense training meals. A person can eat anytime that is convenient to him/her. But people who undergo HIIT are advised to eat healthy carbohydrates and natural sugars.

High intensity trainers are given advice to take protein shakes, smoothies or fruit & vegetable juices for added nutrition.

Chapter 8: Mix Hiit Workouts

The best way to optimize your HIIT program is to mix intensity interval running, cycling, and bodyweight workouts. There's nothing wrong with focusing on just one, but if you aim to lose weight faster, then it's best to alternate these three exercises every week.

You'll also get a full fitness workout with all three. Focusing on just one will limit the development of your body to only a selected muscle group. Losing weight is inevitable, but muscle strength and toning will not be distributed evenly. If you mix all three, however, you are sure to not only shed fats, but also improve your cardio, optimize endurance, and gain strength.

Furthermore, as discussed earlier, doing the same routine for two consecutive days won't give the desired effect. Since these three focus on different muscle groups, you can exercise daily. Exerting effort everyday will make your body cry out those fats, so you double the results in the same amount of time as with the other programs.

Training Schedule

The routines explained in the previous chapters will come to play in this program. You may have noticed by now that the running, cycling and bodyweight programs were simply combined to create the ultimate HIIT 7-week workout.

Generally, beginners can start directly with this program, but it is highly advised that they further lower the intensity of bodyweight exercises. However, if you have experience with other fitness programs, you are free to follow this training schedule.

	Mon	Tue	Wed	Thu	Fri	Sat	Sun
Week 1	BW Level 1	Run Level 1	Cycle Level 1	BW Level 1	Run Level 1	Rest	Stretch
Week 2	Run Level 1 Increased sprint time	BW Level 1 Increased Reps	Cycle Level 2	BW Level 1 Increased Reps	Run Level 1 Increased sprint time	Rest	Stretch
Week	BW	Run	BW	Cycl	BW	Rest	Stretch

k 3	Level 2	Level 2	Level 2	e Level 2 With 135 RPM	Level 2	st	h
Week 4	Cycle Level 3	BW Level 2 Increased rounds	Run Level 2 With incline	BW Level 2 Increased rounds	Cycle Level 3 With 140 RPM	Rest	Stretch
Week	BW Level 3	Run Level 3	BW Level 3	Cycle Level	BW Level 3	Rest	Stretch

5				l 3 With 140 RPM			
Week 6	Run Level 3 With incline	BW Level 3	Cycle Level 4	BW Level 3 Decreased time	Run Level 3 With incline	Rest	Stretch
Week 7	BW Level 3 Decreased time	Cycle Level 4 With 115	BW Level 3 Decreased time	Run Level 3 With incline	BW Level 3 Decreased time	Rest	Stretch

		RPM				

Reminders and Tips

Just like the training schedule, the reminders for this program are the combination of the previously discussed trainings. There are, however, some additional information and tips you have to know before diving in the workout.

If you are a beginner, and you have more than 50 pounds to lose to reach your target, you are encouraged to start with the running HIIT program. Progress to the cycling HIIT program upon completion of the first one, and afterwards, to the bodyweight exercises HIIT program. Once you've completed the training of all three, you are free enjoy the mix HIIT program. This framework will allow your body to gradually adjust to intense physical activities. Another advantage of following this sequence is that your body will be at a constant shock, hence you will continuously lose weight even after your tenth or fifteenth week of exercising.

Basic yoga is highly recommended as your Sunday activity for this program. If classes are out of the question, you can simply download workout videos and follow them at home.

Lastly, for optimum results, don't forget to supplement this program with proper diet. Your metabolism may improve dramatically, but this doesn't mean you're free to eat huge amounts of whatever. Stick to healthy choices and stay away from junk food as much as you can.

Chapter 9: Getting Started

HIIT exercises are beneficial, but you should take note that they may also have certain disadvantages. For instance, they have a higher risk of cardiac events and musculoskeletal injury. Nonetheless, HIIT has been studied as a training method for individuals with congestive heart failure and heart disease. The participants of the study were able to tolerate high intensity intervals without experiencing any negative effects.

What's more, the participants experienced a lot of improvements in their cardiovascular function as compared to the participants who performed continuous moderately intense training. So is HIIT safe? Well, it may or may not be safe for you. As mentioned in the previous chapter, it is crucial to seek medical advice before you follow an HIIT exercise program.

Safety Concerns With Regard to HIIT Training

Obese individuals and people who have been sedentary or inactive for a long period of time may be at risk of coronary disease. Likewise, those who have a history of diseases, such as diabetes and hypertension, may not be allowed to partake in an HIIT exercise program. People whose cholesterol levels are not normal as well as those who smoke cigarettes frequently are also at risk of coronary disease.

Anyone with a health condition is advised to obtain medical clearance before going on HIIT training. In addition, those who plan to do HIIT should establish a good level of fitness. They need to have a base fitness level, so they will not experience any health issues. A base fitness level is generally consistent aerobic training for a few weeks and results in muscular adaptations.

Muscular adaptations can improve the ability of your body to transport oxygen to your muscles. You can perform this aerobic training three to five times per week for twenty to sixty minutes per session with a moderately hard intensity. You need to establish the right muscle strength and exercise form before you engage in regular HIIT, so you can reduce your risk of musculoskeletal injury.

It is very important for you to modify the intensity of your work interval to your preferred level. This is so you will not experience discomfort or pain, and you can avoid injury. Everyone, regardless of gender, fitness level, and age, should follow this protocol. Safety should be your main priority all the time. Also, you should concentrate more on finding your own optimal training intensity as opposed to keeping up with other people.

How to Get Started

In order for you to get started with your HIIT program, you should select an aerobic exercise, such as stationary bicycling. Do not forget to warm up before exercising as well as cool down afterwards in order to avoid injury. You can warm up for five minutes before performing several alternating recovery and speed intervals. Three to four of each interval is sufficient.

For example, you can warm up for five minutes with three to four levels of exertion. You can take a minute for speed with seven to nine levels of exertion, and then two minutes for recovery with five to six levels of exertion. You can have another minute for speed with five to six levels of exertion and another couple of minutes for recovery with five to six levels of exertion.

Finally, you can take one minute for speed with seven to nine levels of exertion, two minutes for recovery with five to six levels of exertion, and five minutes for cool down with three to four levels of exertion. Your total time for these series of exercises is twenty-two minutes.

The protocols for HIIT can vary. There is not really just one way to structure HIIT exercises. Hence, you can experiment with longer and shorter speed and recovery intervals. Find whatever works well for you. You can work your way up to eight to ten speed intervals gradually if you want. See to it that you consider your fitness goals when you exercise.

The most common mistake that people have with regard to interval training is that they fail to have sufficient recovery intervals. It is encouraged that you do HIIT exercises one to two times per week. Do not attempt to perform HIIT exercises more than this in order to reduce your chances of having an injury.

HIIT is a high intensity training method that is best used periodically for about six weeks to enhance regular training. It is not ideal to be used for a year or so. If you wish to achieve best results, you should work with a fitness trainer who can give you a personalized training plan.

With regard to diet, you should carefully watch what you eat. Stick to lean meat for your source of protein, and do not overindulge in carbs and sugar. See to it that you have a balanced diet. Do not rely too much on protein shakes, bars, and supplements. It is a good idea to plan your meals ahead, so you can save time.

Carbohydrates, in the form of whole grains, are recommended to give your body the energy it needs. You should eat before and after you work out. You need carbohydrates to carry protein to your muscles. You can have twenty to twenty-five grams of protein and forty to fifty grams of carbohydrates within one to two hours of working out.

If you like dairy, do not worry because you can still have Greek yogurt and fat-free milk. Drinking milk after a workout is actually a great way to recover. Dairy is a good source of leucine, an amino acid that is responsible for increasing your strength. Dairy also has calcium, vitamin D, and whey protein, which are effective in decreasing body fat and maintaining body mass.

It is ideal that you eat five small meals per day instead of three large ones. This is so you can boost your metabolism faster. You will also not get hungry often throughout the day if you eat five small meals. You can even have cheat days while on your HIIT program. This will allow your taste buds to have a break.

However, you should be consistent with your schedule and eating patterns. You can choose a cheat snack per day, a cheat meal per week, or a specific cheat day for your food cravings. Do not choose all three randomly because this can only lead to weight gain. Do not overestimate how much exercise you can do to burn off the calories.

Chapter 10: Planning The Timing Of Your High-Intensity Interval Workout

The timing you assign to your workouts is extremely important. As a starter, you may want to start small. Your workout should be between 15 to 30 minutes long. The short resting periods are not included in this count. If your exercises are picked well, you are not likely to get to thirty minutes on your first few attempts. You should have 7 cardio exercises, three upper-body workouts, three lower-body exercises, and two core exercises. This routine is the best for losing weight. In your plan, schedule your exercises. Your schedule should be something similar to-

4 cardio workouts

2 upper-body workouts

2 lower-body workouts

2 core workout

1 upper-body workout

1 lower-body workout

3 cardio workouts

The schedule above is only a suggestion. It is a workout schedule that I found works for me. If you find a schedule that works better for you, switch it. This type of routine is perfect for losing weight.

When you decide on your exercise schedule, you can go on to assign the time to each exercise group. Decide on how many minutes you expect your first session to be. The best way to schedule your workout and rest is exercising for twenty minutes and resting for ten. However, when I started high-intensity interval workouts, I did not make it to twenty minutes before finding that I could not move. And so, I designed another schedule. This schedule consisted of a 15-minute work out followed by a 5-7 minute rest session. This was the schedule I started with. As I improved, I moved on to the 'twenty-minute workout session followed by a ten-minute short resting period. Remember that if you are going for a twenty-minute workout session, your short resting period is not included in the twenty minutes.

One mistake some beginners make is not allocating enough rest time. You should have short resting periods compulsorily. The short resting periods in high-intensity interval workouts are mandatory. The short resting periods are the intervals. They are mandatory and even feature in the workouts name- High-Intensity **Interval** Training. It is the short resting periods and interval that allow the workout to be effective. The short resting periods allow your heart rate to increase. They also cause an increase in blood lactate, blood circulation, and muscle lactate. With this in mind, you can now create a workout to suit you. During the rest period, you can either cool down by stretching each muscle or by full body stretches.

One thing I noticed was that I had trouble sticking to the time when I became more tired. As I grew more tired, I started to slow down and so, a workout I planned for two minutes ended up taking two minutes and twenty seconds If you find this happening, it is relatively normal. The solution is to push as hard as you can. Ignore the screaming in your limbs and the pain everywhere. Push as hard as you can. A trainer I met once said she encouraged people in her class to either concentrate entirely on the workout or chant encouragement to themselves while they workout. I have also found out that music helps. Get a good workout song if you think it will help. With this combination, losing weight is a lot much easier.

HIGH-INTENSITY INTERVAL TRAINING, HYDRATION AND DIET

People often wonder if one should be taking water during high-intensity interval training. The answer is yes. Staying hydrated is extremely important for a good exercise session. Few things are worse than getting parched while exercising. Drink water before, during and after your high-intensity interval training exercises. Do you know that water has zero calories?

Drinking water also aids metabolism. This means it can actually help in losing weight. As a plus, you can mix glucose in your water for energy, or grab an energy drink.

The only thing one must be careful of is the amount. You should take small sips. I found that gulping down water gave me cramps if I exercise soon after. For this reason, you should be well hydrated hours before you start your high-intensity interval training. As a matter of fact, you should always be well hydrated.

A common question asked by people interested in losing weight is if they should combine their HIIT exercises with diets. The short answer is yes but it is not that simple. A good diet is always a plus. However, if you are going to do high-intensity interval training, you should be on a well-planned diet. A diet is not the same as starving one's self. The difference is that in a diet, the person interested in losing weight concentrates on eating only for the purpose of absorbing needed nutrients. The person has to cut down on calories and carbs.

In actual fact, to lose weight, I was on a diet and engaged in high-intensity interval training thrice in a week. If you are going to embark on high-intensity interval training for the purpose of losing weight, you should be watching what you are eating anyway. Do not mar your progress by concentrating on burning calories, increasing metabolism and losing weight while going ahead to consume unhealthy amounts of calories. If you are embarking on high-intensity interval training, at the very least, you should be calorie watching.

Chapter 11: Sample Workout

The following sample workout program is ideal because anyone qualified for HIIT can do it. That's because it doesn't require a fitness coach or any equipment. But if you have the equipment, you can go ahead and use it. The important thing is that you get the basics down. It's simple enough but there's no sacrifice of effectiveness.

The program consists of:

- ☐ 1 minute of sprinting or fast jogging
- ☐ 2 minutes of slow jogging or walking

That would be your alternating work and recovery intervals. You can see that it follows the 1:2 ratio described in the previous chapter. Depending on your current condition, you can do this in 5-10 cycles every session and adjust accordingly if you are having trouble. Because this only involves only running and jogging, you can do this in an elliptical, on a treadmill, or anywhere outside.

Progression

If you just do the above sample over and over again, you'll find that it will get easier. When that point comes, you'll know that you're no longer gaining anything. Thus, progression is important. Here is a sample progression you can follow spread across 8 weeks.

Week 1:

- Warm up = 5 Minutes

- Intense Interval = 1 Minute

- Recovery Interval = 2 Minutes

- Cycles (Repetitions) = 2 times

- Cool Down = 5 Minutes

Week 2:

- Warm up = 5 Minutes
- Intense Interval = 1 Minute
- Recovery Interval = 2 Minutes
- Cycles (Repetitions) = 3 times
- Cool Down = 5 Minutes

Week 3:

- Warm up = 5 Minutes
- Intense Interval = 1 Minute
- Recovery Interval = 2 Minutes
- Cycles (Repetitions) = 4 times
- Cool Down = 5 Minutes

Week 4:

- Warm up = 5 Minutes

- Intense Interval = 1 Minute 30 seconds

- Recovery Interval = 3 Minutes

- Cycles (Repetitions) = 2 times

- Cool Down = 5 Minutes

Week 5:

- Warm up = 5 Minutes

- Intense Interval = 1 Minute 30 seconds

- Recovery Interval = 3 Minutes

- Cycles (Repetitions) = 3 times

- Cool Down = 5 Minutes

Week 6:

- Warm up = 5 Minutes

- Intense Interval = 1 Minute 30 seconds

- Recovery Interval = 3 Minutes
- Cycles (Repetitions) = 4 times
- Cool Down = 5 Minutes

Week 7:

- Warm up = 5 Minutes
- Intense Interval = 2 Minutes
- Recovery Interval = 4 Minutes
- Cycles (Repetitions) = 3 times
- Cool Down = 5 Minutes

Week 8:

- Warm up = 5 Minutes
- Intense Interval = 2 Minutes
- Recovery Interval = 4 Minutes
- Cycles (Repetitions) = 4 times
- Cool Down = 5 Minutes

When you finish this 8-week run of the program, you can adjust according to your capabilities, goals, or both. Increase the duration of intervals, add cycles, or both.

Once you start, you may find that this schedule can be too hard or too easy. If you are having such trouble with the durations in the high intensity intervals, know that you can adjust them to fit your abilities and goals.

As you go along, you can replace the exercises with your preference. For example, if you have an exercise bike, you can pedal instead of running/jogging/walking. Do some fast pedaling for the high intensity periods. Then, do some slow to moderate pedaling for the recovery periods.

Lastly, doing HIIT does not mean in any way that you need to give up all other aerobic exercises. You can balance them out. The key here is moderation. To gain the benefits, you should challenge yourself but not to the point that you bring yourself to the ground.

Chapter 12: Ways To Implement The Law Of Attraction

"The brain is such a transmitter & receiver of vibrational energy." – Albert Einstein

Two famous scientists "Albert Einstein" & "Thomas Alva Edison" have successfully proved the above statement with their experiments. Our school textbooks have taught us – "Each cell in our human body simply transmits energy." But as we grow up, we forget the basic law of the universe & get lost with such a series of negative emotions. Every single thing on this planet is really made up of atoms that comprise of – protons, electrons & neutrons. The negatively charged particles of the atoms that're known as electrons are simply made up of vibration, energy & frequency. Everything on this planet has vibrations. The most magical organ of our body, the brain – can easily create any frequency with our thought processes & emotions that in turn have the power to affect the physical matter.

"You simply get what you think about most of the time" – This famous quote by Earl Nightingale is what the law of attraction is all about. Like attracts like, vibrations simply attract similar vibrations, the closer the vibration is, the stronger is the magnetic pull. Knowing what you actually want, feeling the burning desire to attain it & the belief that you're worthy of it makes the law of attraction work in every facet of your life.

Efforts to make law of attraction work

You can easily manifest your way to achieving success, love, money, relationship, abundance & happiness in a short period if you start believing & getting yourself into action. The following steps set out below can really help you to make the law of attraction work in your life:

Affirmations

The best way to influence your subconscious mind & manifest your desires in your entire life is through affirmations. Write strong positive affirmations & read them regularly on a constant basis. Create your own list of affirmations based on your desires & goals & just read them aloud as often as possible.

" i'll definitely be able to just make a career of my passion, & I know the universe will actually attract the abundance & manifest the success I need."

What're you waiting for? Write something similar to the one above based on your desires & start reading your affirmation on such a regular basis.

Faith

Repeating your affirmations & positive thoughts, again & again, will actually help to increase the faith you've in your desires. When your thoughts & faith combine, the subconscious mind acknowledges these positive vibrations & transmits them directly to the universe.

Start using your faith in the right way & stop those unnecessary fears, doubts & negative emotions from entering all of your thought patterns.

Visualize

Visualizing is really the best positive way

to just prepare your mind to get rid of those unnecessary negative thoughts. When you simply visualize your desires, they become burning desires, & you can see them happening in your whole mind in the form of imagination.

Imagine yourself sitting in the car you always wanted to buy. Experience the interior design of the car, feel it & visualize your emotions when you first put your foot on the accelerator. When you simply keep doing this on such a regular basis more often than not, you attract your desire & make it into reality.

Gratitude

Let's say you've put in so much effort to just make that special handmade diary with such a list of beautiful memories for your friend's birthday & all you receive is a "Thank you" with no emotion. You definitely won't be making the same effort for his next birthday. Instead, if the friend expresses his appreciation to the gift with enthusiasm, you'll get excited & give him such a special gift again.

The universe also acts in the same way – when you just express gratitude to the universe for all the good things you have, then the universe will also just be giving you better things if you're open to receive them with equal appreciation. Write a gratitude list & keep adding more to the list whenever you're happy with certain things or situations. This simple exercise will elevate your mood & make your mind shift to the things that'll make you happier.

Board of dreams or visions
How awesome would it be if you simply got to see your visions in the form of images every single day? Dream boards or vision boards are the most popular

exercise you can do, which basically help you to understand the depth of your desires & what you really want from them. These boards can have images or wordings connected to your desire.

You can easily create your own vision board or dream board by collecting pictures from the magazines or the Internet, which are actually linked to your desires & paste them onto the board. You can even add writings or quotes or affirmations to the board. Keep this board in a place where you can easily see it every day & read out the affirmations or quotes as often as possible. Images simply serve as a reminder of your desire & whenever you see these, you remind yourself of what you're trying to attract.

Sensory visualization
Visualizing your desires by utilizing all the senses in your body is called sensory

visualization. When you just recreate your mental, sensory experience of sound, vision, touch, taste & smell, you get to experience those senses. When you really want to manifest love into your entire life, you tend to visualize your dream partner or the person whom you're attracted to. Let it not be an image, simply make it a sensory visualization by imagining how it feels when you just hug or kiss your partner.

Loosen yourself & feel free
Are you constantly worrying about what people will simply think about you? Is your action based on what society will think? Do you really get more conscious of your emotions when you're around people? If you've answered positively to all the above questions, then it's time for you to just let yourself flow in a freer manner. A simple exercise should do the trick.

Get to the comfort zone of your room, switch on that favorite meaningful music, dance or sing like nobody is watching. Loosen your whole body, feel the flow of the energy within yourself, release all the tensions & enjoy that moment. This final step will actually help you to overcome your own restrictions & make you feel more positive & confident. Staying grounded & living in this moment is what's important.

Try this simple exercise!

- Jot down the list of things you desire.
- Rate them in the range of 0-10. The rating should be simply based on the belief you've in manifesting the respective desire.
- Once you've prioritized your desires based on your belief, start writing such a list of affirmations for them on a chart paper.

- Take a board, pin the paper where you've mentioned the desire, fix the chart paper which has the list of affirmations, try getting photos or images which are just in some way connected to your desires & paste them onto the board.
- Once the board, i.e., vision board, is ready, place it in such a location where you can see it every day.
- Look at the images & visualize them often. Read those affirmations aloud whenever you can. Connect yourself to the vision,

When you just keep doing this repeatedly, the belief in your whole desire increases & you start loving your visions & take the necessary steps to simply make them happen. By believing in your vision, you just take responsibility for your life & your entire perception towards life changes as you realize that you've the power & energy to change your thoughts & start manifesting all the things you may really want in your entire life.

Chapter 13: Nutrition With Hiit

To get the best results with H IIT, having a thought out nutrition plan will ensure that most benefits. The body needs to have enough glycogen to get through the high-intensity level intervals. In addition, hydration is incredibly important.

To prepare the body for the HIIT workout, a pre-workout meal is also essential. You should eat 2 to 3 hours before your workout and include fruit carbs and protein. Carbs will help you with the energy burst necessary for your workout to be most effective.

You do not need to eliminate any particular types of food, either. Using protein only, as some weight loss plans is not recommended, as it doesn't provide enough fuel. Of course you want to have protein, but during a workout, carbs are more beneficial. You can use carbs, very efficiently and effectively, so you don't want to cut them out of your diet.

Dairy has also been found to build muscle mass and decrease fat because of the calcium, vitamin D and protein. If you are lactose intolerant, there are a number of protein drinks available that you can have which could be considered a milk or a protein-based drink. Having something like this after your workout will help with your recovery.

Drinking plenty of water will help you flush out any toxins and HIIT requires lots of fluids. If you drink at least eight glasses of water a day, you will stay hydrated. Nutritional supplements are not necessary when you first get started with H IIT.

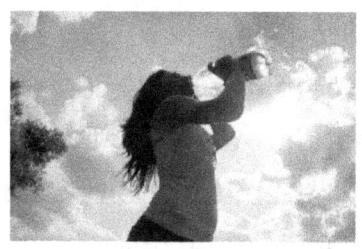

Fruit, vegetables, lean protein, carbohydrates and good fats are a strong diet for effective workouts. Because HIIT is burning carbs effectively, you can test how many carbs you'll need in your daily diet to see what works for you.

Many higher-level athletes do use protein supplements to increase endurance during workouts that are high-intensity.

These are usually consumed before you start working out. Another supplement that is popular, which helps minimize muscle fatigue, is beta alanine, an amino acid. In addition, after workout many athletes will have an additional protein supplement to provide energy and keep burning fat after the workout. However, this is not something you necessarily need to get started with the right way you can wait until you've built up some endurance and have adjusted your diet for the best benefits.

Chapter 14: Recovering From Hiit

Considering HIIT is a very intense workout, it is absolutely vital that we take proper recovery into account as well. HIIT should only be done 2 times a week; 3 times as a maximum. These HIIT days should always be staggered and HIIT should never be done on back to back days. One of the reasons for this is because how taxing HIIT is on our muscles. With any sort of training, muscles are broken down. After they repair is when they get stronger, but if we don't give them the proper time to recover from something as intense as HIIT, we will see a dip in our results. This can also lead to over training of the body, which causes the following symptoms: increased irritability, fatigue, interrupted sleep, and other symptoms that are all a sign of overtraining.

It is important for recovery that we first follow the basics of recovery. These basics include getting proper nutrition and getting the proper amount of sleep. Before a HIIT workout take into consideration what you are going to do for the workout. Considering all HIIT workouts include a tearing down of the muscles it is absolutely imperative that we provide the means for the muscle to recover! This would mean that we need to eat foods that are high in protein to aid in muscle recovery. Not only that, but most HIIT workouts utilize the use of cardio in the routine as well. For intense cardio sessions it is also very important that we have carbs that will properly fuel us to get through these cardio sessions. So not only should we eat food that is high in protein but high in carbs as well. Considering every workout will be intense I would recommend eating complex carbs that are also high in protein. Foods rich in complex carbs would include: pastas, greens, beans, potatoes, oatmeal and the like. It is recommended that you fuel up two hours before your actual workout to reduce the chance of cramping.

Not only is eating the proper fuel to get your workout going important, it is also vital that we sleep the proper amount every night. With proper sleep comes greater muscle repair and recovery. The recommended amount of sleep in a healthy adult is seven to nine hours, but professional athletes (The proprietors of this type of training) typically spend eight to ten hours a night sleeping for recovery. Once you start this type of training, as a rule of thumb it is best to sleep seven to nine hours. If you are feeling overly taxed it would be wise to even add in some extra sleep as well. This sleep can be tacked on to your nightly rest or even come in the form of an afternoon nap if you so desire. Stay away from sleep aids and other forms of drugs to achieve the amount of sleep you need because those significantly lower your sleep quality causing the recovery you receive from sleep to be reduced.

Another great way to recover from doing HIIT is by adding in a stretching after your workout. Stretching is an effective cool down which will help your body tremendously. Without proper stretching techniques you risk leaving your muscles in flexion which can lead to you being very tight and stiff and more prone to injury. Stretching also improves blood flow to stretched areas and this blood flow provides a flushing out of lactic acid. Lactic acid is what causes muscle soreness and muscle tightness. With a reduced amount of that you will be feeling your workout a lot less the next day. Stretching also helps with mobility. Mobility is important to reduce aches and pains but also to improve the amount of work that your muscles are doing. The lower you can go in a squat the more muscle that will be worked.

The final method of recovery that will be discussed is the use of SMR techniques. SMR stands for Self-Myofascial Release. This technique includes the use of a foam roller and using your body weight on top of the foam roller to break up restricted tough connective tissue. SMR has been proven to increase athletic performance, reduce pain, and even encourages soft tissue repair. Not only that, but this technique can also improve flexibility as well. Using a combination of stretching and foam rolling would be the most effective way to recover from doing HIIT. Also taking into account proper nutrition and proper sleep as well.

Chapter 15: Enzyme Adaptation

In reviewing the three energy pathways, I mentioned key enzymes involved in those processes. At this point we can start looking at the enzyme adaptations that take place in the human body during high intensity interval training. In this lesson, I give an overview of enzyme adaptation and in the following three lessons, I'll supply information about specific and relevant enzyme adaptations that are connected to HIIT.

It is well documented that aerobic training protocols will increase oxidative enzyme activity but will not affect glycolytic enzymes. To influence the anaerobic metabolic enzymes the intensity has to be acceptable. In studies where the intensity has been around 60–70% of the absolute maximal velocity, there has been no increase in anaerobic metabolism. To affect the anaerobic metabolism the intensity has to be at least 80–90% of maximal velocity.

The activity of glycolytic and oxidative enzymes has not been shown to increase in well-trained individuals and athletes who participate in HIIT. The reason is that they may already have high levels of glycolytic and oxidative enzyme activities.

This is in contrast to the untrained person, where most types of metabolic stress may lead to oxidative adaptations. The increased enzyme activity in people just starting to exercise may be related to their lower levels of enzyme activity in general. Basically since the untrained person is more or less starting from zero when they start exercising, it makes sense that they would experience measurable increases in their enzyme activity.

The Big Takeaway

•By understanding how the body and its enzyme adaptations respond to certain HIIT workouts, you can design HIIT workouts that will provide both health benefits and an engaging experience for your clients. You won't have to design workouts that only leave clients exhausted and lying on the floor because you'll have a better understanding of how less intense, more varied HIIT routines, that don't leave people depleted, can also greatly benefit their health and fitness.

•Second, intensity matters when it comes to enzyme adaptation.

•Third, when it comes to more experienced clients, then you have to be more specific in the HIIT workout design to achieve enzyme adaptation.

- Fourth, in order to enhance the activity of enzymes, the HIIT protocol has to produce high metabolic flux through relevant pathways or transport systems. For example, to increase the activity of the ATP-CP system, we need to utilize short work duration protocols with long rest duration.

Chapter 16: Home Hiit Exercises

There are many movements you can do at home for HIIT. If you have cardio equipment, right off the bat you have a great tool for high intensity interval training. HIIT can be done on any cardio equipment. In fact, for obese and very poorly conditioned individuals, cardio equipment makes a wise choice for mode, especially pedalling devices.

Here are additional movements for HIIT (this list isn't complete; the variety of moves is almost endless). To manipulate intensity, go faster or slower, higher, farther, deeper or more shallow, and/or hold light hand weights. You'll see that some of the moves are geared towards more experienced trainees and some towards novices and the very poorly conditioned:

Squat Jump

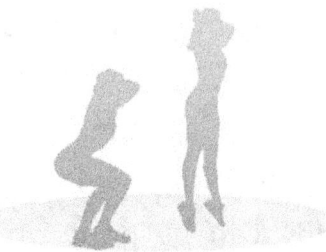

Lower into a squat, then jump off the floor. Land into the squat and repeat.

Tuck Jump

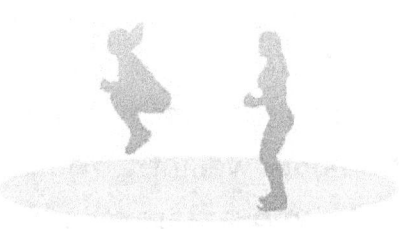

Jump and tuck legs/knees under you as much as possible.

Bench Hop

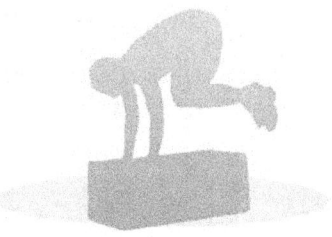

Avoid the cheat move of taking a "baby" hop before the main hop.

Box Jump

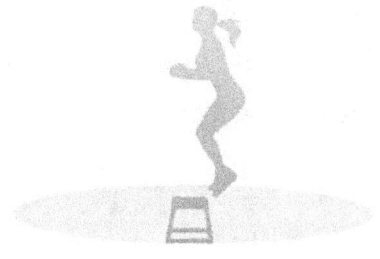

Use a sturdy exercise box or "plyometric stool." Jump up and down, landing with both feet at once at all times. **Variation:** straddle jump.

Box scissor jump

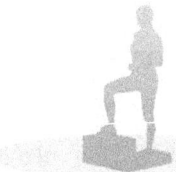

Begin with right foot on box, left on floor. Then quickly switch feet so that right foot is on floor, left foot on box. A variation is to tap ball of foot to box:

Floor skater jump

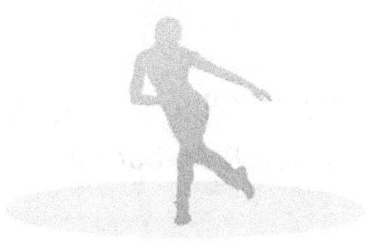

From a partial squat position, lower deeper and extend right foot out to the side, then bring foot back to original position and simultaneously extend left foot out to the side.

Floor scissor jump (jump lunge)

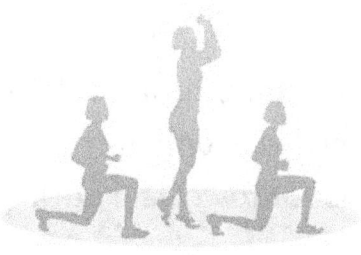

Start in a lunge position. Jump, switch legs in the air and land. Go back and forth.

Lateral jump

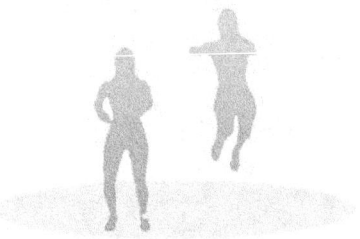

Feet together, jump from side to side. Increase intensity by jumping over a height or a width (mat or towel laid out).

Burpee

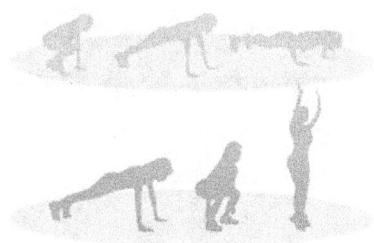

Drop into a full squat, palms on floor. Thrust legs out behind you so that you're in the top of a pushup, then bring legs back under you, spring up and raise hands overhead.

Mountain climber

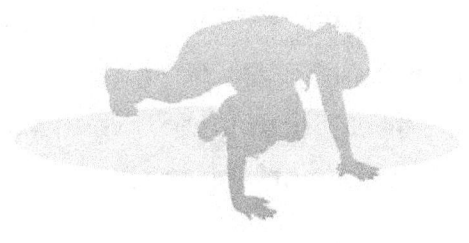

Get into a top push up, then bring knees to chest, alternating legs. Variation: Place hands on edge of sturdy table (high modified push up position).

Chair squat

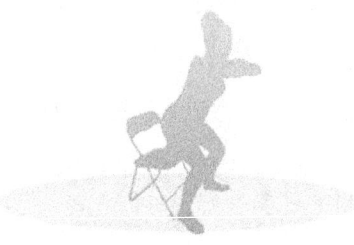

Use a sturdy seat or medium size exercise box/stool. Space feet shoulder width apart while seated, then stand. Sit and stand as fast as you can. Tip: Do not lift or rock any part of the feet off the floor when you sit! Try to keep hands off the seat.

Bodyweight half squat

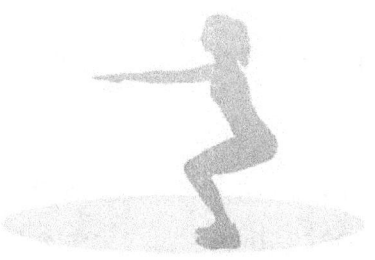

Sink down so that thighs are parallel to floor.

Chapter 17: More On Hiit Nutrition

There is no single set-in-stone rule of exactly **what** should be eaten pre- and post-HIIT.

Pre-workout: Some people do well with a little fruit before the session. Others do well with yogurt or pure protein pre-workout. However, we can all agree that a large meal soon before exercise, or a junk food item, is not a smart plan.

Some do well doing HIIT first thing in the morning without any food, in a fasted state. Some other trainees "need" to eat something soon before the workout, while still others are okay eating a little something one or two hours prior to the session.

The rules change if you have diabetes, but in general, there's no medical reason why you should eat soon before HIIT unless you've found that HIIT on an empty stomach leads to queasiness or light-headedness.

It boils down to what works best for you. This includes hydration. Some trainees will get a cramp without it; while others don't want to have to empty their bladder in the middle of a HIIT session, and therefore won't hydrate prior or even during.

Post-workout. Here is where things get interesting. Post-HIIT, your body is in a huge state of oxygen debt, when glucose metabolism is at its finest hour. Your body needs lots of carbohydrates to aid in recovery, and protein (about 20 grams will suffice). Plus water. Drink up.

This is the time where, if you planned on eating a brownie or ice cream that day, it should be done right after HIIT, as your body will utilize more of the carbs and calories for recovery at this critical time.

But this doesn't mean you **should** eat junk food post-HIIT. It only means if you're planning on eating junk or indulgence-type food (like lasagne, roast beef and gravy, and control the portion!) at some point in the week, try to schedule it for right after HIIT.

Otherwise, a good post-workout meal would be a full meal that should be plant based, such as around four ounces of poultry, fish or grass fed beef, a green salad and a serving of a complex carbohydrate: rice, barley, potatoes, lentils or quinoa, for instance.

Or, you can have a large fruit plate with cottage cheese, or a large glass of juice with some protein. A fruit smoothie with some chicken salad would be good as well.

Avoid the so-called "sports drinks." These often amount to being no more than liquid candy with some minerals tossed in. Milk is a much better post-workout beverage than some neon-coloured drink. Never **not** consume anything after HIIT.

Chapter 18: Catecholamines Response To Sprint Interval Training

The catecholamines include noradrenaline, adrenaline, and dopamine. These hormones and neurotransmitters play an essential role in the metabolic, cardiovascular, and immune systems. High intensity activities with short recovery periods have been shown to increase the concentration of catecholamines in the plasma. Therefore, catecholamines influence the body's metabolic responses to exercise in an overwhelmingly positive way.

Dr. Richard Bracken at Swansea University examined the influence of sprint interval training on this catecholamine response.[33] He and his team established a sprint interval protocol consisting of ten rounds of 6-second maximal-effort sprints, followed by 30 seconds of rest, hence a work-to-rest ratio of 1:5. The result: the plasma concentration of noradrenaline increased 14.5-fold from baseline to post-exercise levels. Plasma adrenaline levels increased 6.3-fold during the protocol. The protocol was not found to have any influence on dopamine.

Other results from this study showed that heart rate progressively increased during the 10 sprints to reach an average peak value of 173 beats per minute. The lactate levels increased to 9.6 mmol, which is a 43-fold increase. These two results indicate that we need to use very high intensity protocols to create high levels of lactate accumulation to influence catecholamine response.

The exercise physiologist E. Gail Trapp and his team at University of New South Wales investigated the catecholamine response to two sprint interval protocols.**34** The first protocol consisted of 60 rounds of 8 seconds of maximal intensity sprinting with each followed by 12 seconds of recovery, so a work-to-rest ratio of 1:1.5. The second protocol consisted of 20 rounds of 24 seconds of sprinting at maximal intensity with each followed by 36 seconds of recovery, so also a work-to-rest ratio of 1:1.5. Both protocols reported increased levels of noradrenaline and adrenaline.

Researchers that have utilized the Wingate protocol (30 seconds of all-out effort, followed by a 4-minute rest, so a work-to-rest ratio of 1:8) have seen an 85% increase in adrenaline concentration and an 88% increase in noradrenaline concentration.

The Big Takeaway

- First, these studies show that high intensity interval training protocols induce significant increases in plasma catecholamines.

- Second, catecholamine concentration is closely related to exercise intensity.

- Third, HIIT is an effective training method for fat loss. Why? Because adrenaline, one of the catecholamines that HIIT protocols increase the levels of, increases lipolysis, which is the breakdown of fats in the body. We'll discuss fat loss and HIIT more in the next lesson.

HIIT and Fat Oxidation

Let me start with this encouraging news: it has been shown that people that are engaged in intense or vigorous activities are leaner than those involved in less intense activities.[35]

While, so far in Section I, I haven't focused directly on fat oxidation, meaning the burning of fat to fuel the body, if you look at the adaptations that take place during HIIT, you notice how effective it is at this. For example, in Lesson 10, we learn how HIIT will increase the activity of the mitochondrial enzyme citrate synthase. Let me add here that the increase of this enzyme leads to fat oxidation. So, it is time that we concentrate strictly on HIIT and fat loss, something that we can already predict that most people at any level of fitness are very interested in.

There are many possible mechanisms stemming from HIIT that promote fat loss. In "The Big Takeaway" of the previous lesson, I pointed out the effect of HIIT on catecholamine response. Adrenaline and noradrenaline, two hormones that HIIT increases the levels of in the body, both promote lipolysis, i.e., fat oxidation.

(Because the lipolysis process is a complicated one, like all metabolic processes in the human body, I'm not going to give a full explanation of it in this book.)

Let's start by looking at a 1994 study that is probably the most cited one on HIIT and fat loss. This study, conducted by Professor Angelo Tremblay and his team at Laval University, compared the impact of a HIIT protocol and a steady-state endurance protocol on body fat levels and skeletal muscle metabolism.**36** The study's steady-state group performed 30–45 minutes of continuous cycling, four to five times per week, for 20 weeks. The HIIT group performed 25 sessions of 30 minutes of continuous exercise at 70% of maximum heart rate; and during those 30 minutes, participants also performed 19 short (15–30 seconds) and 16 long (60–90 seconds) interval sessions, over a period of

15 weeks. They completed half of the continuous training session by week five as a preparation for the HIIT sessions. The recovery period between bouts was to allow the heart rate to return to 120–130 beats per minute.

The results: the energy cost, or calories burned, by those in the HIIT group was half of that of those in the steady-state protocol, 57.9 MJ versus 120.4 MJ. This means that the steady-state group burned more calories, about double the amount, than the HIIT group. Now for the amazing part—despite this fact, the reduction of subcutaneous fat was significantly greater in the HIIT group.

Dr. Gail Trapp and his team at University of New South Wales also studied the relationship between HIIT and fat oxidation.[37] This team investigated the response of two sprint interval protocols on glycerol response (we first encountered this study in the previous lesson). The first protocol consisted of 60 rounds of 8 seconds of maximal intensity, followed by 12 seconds of recovery (1:1.5). The second protocol consisted of 20 rounds of 24 seconds of work at maximal intensity, followed by 36 seconds of recovery (1:1.5 again).

The results: there was a significant increase in plasma glycerol concentration, a concentration that could indicate a reliance on burning fats for fuel during exercise. During HIIT's recovery periods, ATP is resynthesized by the aerobic system. Of course, other systems will resynthesize it as well, but if you review the previous lessons on ATP turnover, you will see that the aerobic system will provide greater and greater amounts of energy, as compared to the anaerobic systems, as a HIIT workout progresses.

This happens because of the depletion of phosphocreatine and glycogen, and increases in cytosolic citrate, which inhibits glycolysis. I say all this to explain what HIIT is doing in the body to result in such noticeable fat oxidation.

Another study performed by Dr. Trapp at University of New South Wales was designed to determine the effects of a 15-week HIIT protocol on subcutaneous and trunk fat.**38** The team used two training protocols, one was a steady-state training protocol and the other an 8-second "on" and 12-second "off" (1:1.5) HIIT protocol. The duration of the steady-state protocol was gradually increased to 40 minutes, and the volume of the HIIT protocol reached 60 rounds by the end of the trial period, lasting for 20 minutes total.

The results from this study: significant decreases in total body mass, fat mass

(11.2%), and central abdominal fat (9.5%) occurred in individuals in the HIIT group, but no changes were observed in these areas in the people in the steady-state protocol. Wow—isn't that a win-win for people doing HIIT? They only have to give 20 minutes to a HIIT session to achieve measurable fat loss! Talk about fun on the journey and a fabulous destination all rolled into one!

The Big Takeaway

• First, this should come as no surprise that HIIT is a very effective training method to stimulate fat loss.

• Second, even with the findings in the above studies, we should not totally exclude endurance training because endurance training can help to increase the overall amount of calories burned, and it can also be used to prevent overtraining which can happen with HIIT due to HIIT's intensity.

•Third, a variety of work-to-rest ratios can help stimulate fat loss even more, so don't stick with just one protocol—mix it up and make it fun.

Chapter 19: Hiit For Fat Loss And Muscle Gain

HIIT is no doubt a great way to melt off those body fat. The workout aims at quick fat burning and the ultimate reduction of fat cells that store fat reserves. But before moving on to the mechanism of fat burning by high intensity workouts or any other methods, you need to understand the mechanism of fat storage in the body.

When you consume food, some of it is used as glucose for energy expenditure. The extra food is stored in the form of glycogen in the liver. This is the reserve food that is used once the glucose levels in the body become low.

Fats and triglycerides are also used by the body for energy and fats provide the largest amount of energy. Extra fat is stored in cells called adipocytes that are abundant in the flank, thighs and the abdomen region. The aim of any exercise is to signal the body burn these reserve carbs and fats.

But before this happens, the body has to exhaust the glucose and triglycerides that are already present in the body. Once those are used up for fuel, the body starts to use the reserve glycogen and fats.

How Does HIIT Cause Fat Loss?

Metabolism refers to all the processes that take place in the body. These can be of two types.

- Anabolic

These are the reactions in which new products are synthesized using the reactants that are present in the body. These things are often extracted from the food we take in, such as proteins and carbs.

- Catabolic

These reactions are the ones in which something is broken down into smaller particles or for excretion from the body. These reactions may be fat oxidation in which fats are burnt into their respective components. Other than that, catabolic reactions include carb burning and breaking down of larger nutrients into their monomers use these building blocks for making something new.

Both these reactions take place side by side and both need energy to function. This energy comes from burning carbs that are already present in the body.

When a person performs a high intensity workout, their metabolic rate is enhanced. Due to this acceleration of the metabolic rate, reactions in the body also take place at a faster rate. Since more reactions occur and at a faster rate, the fat reserves in the body also start being used up for energy.

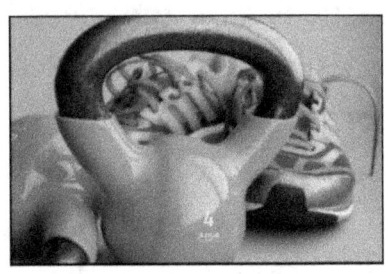

With HIIT your metabolism remains in action even in the resting stage; HIIT is much better at enhancing resting metabolism than aerobic exercises. It keeps the resting metabolism going on at a significant rate for 24 hours after the workout, which is just in time for the next workout. Therefore, it keeps the body burning fat during the whole day, even when at rest.

HIIT And Fat Oxidation

Fat oxidation is the process in which fats are broken down into triglycerides. In cells, oxidation of fat occurs as a result of which triglycerides are produced. These are used for energy provision or they can be stored in the adipose tissue. Since HIIT induces fat oxidation, it ensures that body fat is being broken down instead of getting stored up.

The liver is the only organ in the body that can dispose of cholesterol. When fat reserves build up on the liver, the liver cannot function properly due to pressure exerted on it by the fat concentration. As a result of HIIT, the fat reserves melt which causes the liver to function properly for disposing off cholesterol.

Increase In Growth Hormone Levels

HIIT has also shown to increase growth hormone levels. This hormone is also involved in the fat burning mechanism in the body along with enhancing metabolism. In the presence of this hormone, the metabolic rate of the body improves and the efficiency of metabolism is also enhanced significantly.

During high intensity workouts, a chemical is produced in the body called catecholamine. This chemical facilitates fat loss since it mobilizes the stored fat. The fat reserves keep increasing in the body until the previous ones are burnt.

In the presence of this chemical, the fat that is stored in the adipose tissue is mobilized so that it can be used as fuel for energy. The primary source for fuel in the body is carbohydrates so the body has to produce some kind of chemical to make the fats available for fuel.

How Does HIIT Build Muscle Mass?

HIIT is also responsible for building muscle mass. This is because HIIT builds endurance and causes more blood flow with better contractility to the muscles. The blood carries oxygen and nutrients to all parts of the body. After high intensity workouts, more oxygen is taken to the muscles. This results in oxidative respiration in the muscle.

Anaerobic conditions cause the production of lactic acid in muscles. This is why the muscles feel fatigued and they get sore. If more oxygen is taken to the muscles, aerobic conditions persist and oxidation process occurs. As a result, you build more muscle mass in the long run.

Moreover, blood also takes nutrients to the muscles. These nutrients are essential for the muscle growth and development, especially the proteins. Proteins can be used as energy source for growth of the muscles. Also, they are great for repair.

Every time you work out, muscle wear and tear takes place which has to be treated by the body. Proteins play a role in this process and they repair the muscle fibres that have been damaged during intense workouts. Also, they make new muscle fibres using amino acid as building blocks. These amino acids are used for making muscle proteins called actin and myosin which are responsible for muscle contraction and relaxation.

Metabolism And Muscle Mass

HIIT increases the rate of metabolism in the muscles in active stage and keeps metabolic activities going on even in the resting stage. In the anabolic reactions, new products are made for muscles. In this process, muscle mass is also built. Since high intensity workouts keep the anabolic activities going on for 24 hours following the workout, they ensure that muscle synthesis is taking place at all times.

As such, high intensity workouts are great for burning fat since they increase the metabolic rate and also increase the fat oxidation rate in the body. Plus, it also reduces appetite and increases fat mobility by increasing the amount of catecholamine. Along with fat loss, high intensity workouts are also responsible for increasing lean muscle mass which is a great way for people to get their dream body.

Conclusion

HIIT allows increased weight loss and fitness within a short period of time. However, it is not an easy routine to follow and it cannot be performed by everyone. It requires a fit physique to perform this grueling workout. One can build stamina and endurance gradually by performing HIIT workouts from the beginner level to the advanced level.

With the incorporation of both aerobic and anaerobic components, HIIT really delivers many more benefits than a normal workout routine. However, the intensity of the workout demands care, attention and caution. It's recommended to be incorporated only 2 to 3 times a week. It is also very important to consult a physician to determine whether HIIT is safe for the athlete, as it can result in serious consequences if one's body cannot withstand the strain.

Above all, HIIT is a novel route to fitness. Those in good shape can truly reap the benefits of this routine through a dedicated approach to HIIT.

www.ingramcontent.com/pod-product-compliance
Lightning Source LLC
Chambersburg PA
CBHW071830080526
44589CB00012B/969